Vaccinations and Vaccine Myth Exposed: The reasons to be Afraid

By Daniel Birk

Table of Contents

Introduction

Thank you for your interest in Vaccinations and Vaccination Myths Exposed: the reasons to be Afraid. Vaccinations are a very touchy subject for most, sparking a huge debate and controversy among many. While many are willing to discuss the "positive" impact they have in our lives, nobody wants to discuss an even more serious reality which links Autism to these forced vaccinations. For years both our government and scientists alike have gone back and forth debating the issue of linking vaccines to this illness, but one truth remains, and that is they are harmful and contain large traces of toxins that are harmful to the body.

As you read through this guide you will learn how it came to be that vaccines were created, the effect they've had on our minds and bodies and what to believe as appose to what we are forced to believe. The media as well as doctors portray them as safe and effective, but what goes on behind closed doors that they don't want us to really know? Let's take a further look into the busy world of inoculations.

Chapter 1: The epidemic of Autism

What is Autism and how is it diagnosed?

While there is no clear cut tests to diagnose autism there are many symptoms and signs that can be looked for in both infants and children. Most children who display signs of Autism tend to avoid eye contact, are repetitive in their actions and tend to not respond to their name when called. As the child gets older and is able to verbally communicate better, there are a series of questions that can be asked by a trained professional. Based on the answers the child provides it can be determined whether the child is Autistic or not.

What causes Autism?

Causes and preventive measure

There is no clear answer to the exact route of what causes Autism, but one thing is for sure and that is there is a direct link between it and the chemicals found in vaccines. Originally, it was linked to genetics and an abnormality in the brain yet it was found as early as the forties there was a direct link between the disorder and children getting inoculated. While most try to blame the disease on genetics alone, many doctors recommend a few things to minimize the chances of your child developing Autism in womb.

Take pre-natal vitamins while pregnant

Do not take street drugs or drink while pregnant

Get your vaccines

Depending on medications you took prior to pregnancy, make sure they are approved by your doctor first especially when it comes to epileptic medications.

Autism

A growing epidemic

It is estimated that every 1 in 8 children have been diagnosed with Autism. So what does this mean? Simply put, there is now a 78% increase in children all over the United States being diagnosed with this illness. The question still remains, why is it a growing epidemic and what is causing it? While it's always been known that our government hides behind figures and excuses, Autism seems to become more and more frequent diagnosis the more we press parents and kids in to unnecessary vaccinations.

Chapter 2: Inoculation at an early age

Autism first appeared in cases during 1943. Before 1970, it was estimated that 1 in 10,000 had autism, but by 2008 the number increased to 1 in 150. While we are not only seeing an increase in cases, males are showing to be more likely to develop autism than females with a 4:1 ration. Many suggest an unknown cause behind the epidemic, but one thing remains clear and that's the trend of harmful chemicals such as ethyl mercury and a well-known preservative thimersol. These two well-known components have been used and found in vaccines since 1931. Other known causes behind Autism are not just toxins and deadly chemicals, but live viruses inside them as well.

Centuries back, scientists often injected (infected,) patients with one live virus in order to try and prevent another. In this case the prevention of small pox was created by injecting patients with a live strain of cow pox instead. The first vaccine created was in 1955 for the Polio virus. Later the Diphtheria, Tetanus, and Pertussis were developed during the span from 1906-1946. The DTP combination vaccine was shortly after made available in 1946. It seemed during the following years, scientists would be hard at work creating other vaccines deemed "necessary" including Measles (1969), Mumps (1969),

Pneumonia (1978), and Rubella (1979). During the same year a combination MMR vaccine came to be in which patients were now being given more than vaccine at a time.

Who gets vaccines?

Babies and young kids at risk

It appears that from the time the mother discovers she is pregnant to the many doctor visits that follow, one thing is on every doctor's mind and that is vaccines. During the second trimester, many pregnant mothers are expected to be subjected to various tests and with that comes of course vaccines. Depending on the time of year most OBGYN's will recommend a flu shot as well as a whooping cough vaccination for the mother to be. While you have the choice to fore-go these possibly, unnecessary inoculations, you will again be asked upon the birth of your child.

Typically when a patient refuses a vaccination or decides to "opt-out" they are bombarded with numerous questions from their family physician on the reasons behind their refusal and in some cases even reported to child services after being forced to sign special waiver forms for "child abuse." If that is not enough to scare a patient or parents in to getting these toxic chemicals injected in to their bodies, let the guilt begin! Doctors and pediatricians alike have become notorious for spouting off

5

random numbers and statistics to guilt and scare parents in to conforming to "standard" medical practices which include these harmful vaccinations.

I refused vaccines for my child

What do I do now?

So you've taken a healthier path and decided to not get your child vaccinated, what now right? As mentioned beforehand most doctor offices will require you to sign a waiver that will be retained in your child's medical file. Read the waiver carefully over so you understand what you're being asked to sign. Some parents even go to the extent or crossing out some parts of the forms that they do not agree with and leaves notes of their own before signing and returning the paper. While physicians may claim "by law" you're required to vaccinate your children that simply is not true.

It has become extremely common for parents to take a stance in their children's health and refuse to inoculate. There are many cases where children go to public schools who have not been subjected to the harmful toxins and chemicals and are still allowed to participate just as any other child would. The likely hood of any child catching the disease that's supposed to be prevented is extremely rare and in most cases only exist in slight instances in certain parts of the world.

Chapter 3: Lies and truth perpetuated by the media

How do I know who to believe?

It's no surprise that you'll never hear the same story about anything news worthy from the media twice. While one week they may claim that something is necessary, there will be multiple stories a month later claiming the opposite. It's almost become a game going back and forth between the lies and truth. The media much like our government will tell people whatever they believe they want to hear, and whatever will financially support and over pay the rich.

With all the back and forth between media news outlets it's hard to know who to believe and what to trust, so how do you make your own decision? Remember, it is your life, your family and your right to do what's within the safe realm of care for your children. Refusal to inoculate is neither abuse nor mandated. It is your right as a parent to discover what is and is not right for your child. Always do your homework and look for sources outside the mainstream media for better knowledge and understanding.

One of the biggest lies the media and doctors have told is that those who are not protected against Whooping Cough are the most harmful to your babies and children. Yet when further research was done and real facts were examined, we found the opposite to be true. Children who receive this vaccination are the actual culprits behind this nasty illness. Reason? When your child is vaccinated for this disease, it's actually introducing the virus in to the stream and causing the body's natural immune system to be interfered with and unable to block it naturally.When this happens, a now vaccinated child (who is more likely to get than a non,) gets the illness and thus spreads to other children.

As research has shown over the past years, when the out breaks do occur, it is the non-inoculated children that remain healthier/healthiest whilst those subjected to the vaccines show a high infection rate.

Does the crime fit the punishment?

Laws and penalties for non-vaccinated children

While the rise of non-vaccinated children keeps going, a large public outcry has begun involving parents of vaccinated children. Laws as well as punishments are attempting to be forced upon parents of children who are not vaccinated. We tend to overlook the real issue here. In almost every case where a child is vaccinated against a disease that poses a "threat" to "healthy kids," the real blame lies within those vaccines and the children receiving them.

It's not uncommon to turn on the TV or read in the newspaper how we should have stricter laws or punishments for parents who choose to protect their kids from vaccines. What about those that do vaccinate? As scientists and countless years of research show over and over again, they are spreading all these illnesses. By being injected with these supposed "dead-viruses" we are blocking the body's immune system from doing what it was created to do. Often times the receptors found inside a vaccine, attacks and confuses the natural immune system so when a child does contract the virus its harder or impossible to fight it off.

Symptoms and Side Effects

An over-view of negative side effects involving inoculation

For most parents no matter if they choose to get their child vaccinated in a health clinic or a doctor's office, they are often given hand-outs explaining what the vaccination is for and the health risks involved. Most just accept the papers at face value and still agree to give their child the vaccine and continue on without really reading the side effects or what could happen by putting these chemicals in their bodies. For those who have read the paper, this is some of the things that you can expect to see and have actually been reported as having happened to their children:

Allergic reaction (Swelling, sweating, inability to breathe, loss of color in the face, coughing, fever, and death.)

Fever

On or around injection site (Pain, swelling, redness)

Fatigue

Shivering

Headache

Muscle Pain

Bruising

Abdominal Pain

Diarrhea

Headache

Upper Repertory Infection

Stuffy nose

Sore throat

Blood in Urine or Stool

Pneumonia

Seizures

Inflammation of the stomach or intestines

Vomiting

Fussiness

Non-stop crying

Coma

Permanent brain damage

Loss of appetite

Dizziness/Fainting

Rash

Low platelet count which can then later lead to a blood disorder

Deafness

Pneumonia

While most of these are all symptoms repeated with almost every vaccine, they don't always tell you many of the one's that were listed above. In fact, upon further inspection you will find that beyond rash, redness, fussiness and fatigue they don't really list any other possible symptoms, but do in fact give you a number to call if you lose a loved one from a vaccination related injury or believe your child suffers from an allergic reaction as a result. Still think it's a good idea to vaccinate your child? After all, the media believes the risk of not vaccinating are greater than the side effects of vaccinations. I think most would agree that we enjoy our children happy, alive and well and some things are just not worth the risk of our children's lives. If that's not enough to bother you, let's move on and discuss what exactly are in these vaccinations; chemicals, toxins, and who knows what else.

Chapter 4: Mercury Culprit and Other Ingredients found in Vaccines

During the 80's, the public was introduced into the newest vaccine Hepatitis B and Influenza. By 1991 doctors started to inoculate newborns immediately upon birth with this new Hep B and Flu vaccine. Had this not been enough children started to get this new vaccine as well as DTP vaccines regularly during every doctor visit. All three were known to contain dangerous trace levels up to 125 times their safe level with the dangerous Ethyl Mercury toxins as well as the ever common Thimersol preservative. Due to such high levels of toxicity pregnant mothers were receiving this practice was stopped until the baby was born. In 2002 it was reported that the dangerous preservative Thimersol was removed, but was later discovered to still be found inside these dangerous vaccines.

While the chemicals and preservatives are being allowed to continue so does the number of babies born with Autism and later being diagnosed as children. Meanwhile, no attempts have been made by neither the FDA nor any other organization to remove or alter the chemicals used in vaccines as they have been no known cases that can "directly" correlate autism with the vaccines given.

German scientist Stajich et al did various studies when it came to exposure of mercury after giving preterm infants the hepatitis B vaccine. In 2000 a study was then produced by Pichichero et al claiming that mercury was based on the concentration levels and metabolism of an infant, it would remove itself from their systems naturally following the vaccination. For some time this resolved the idea and threat that Thimerosal was harmful putting the case to rest for a while. Later, in 2005, another study was conducted by researcher Burbacher et al using primates. It was discovered that following an injected, mercury not only lingered, but then traveled to the brain where it was then turned in to mercury chloride. Mercury when received in high enough doses can be extremely dangerous as well have harmful and sometimes lasting effects on not just the human body, but the brain as well.

It's all too well known that every vaccination contains unusually large traces of mercury among other things. So now not only do we have to worry about the side-effects but now were being told that were injecting our children and babies with a harmful chemical known as mercury. There is a vast link connected between the use of mercury and the Autism disease. Ironically, mercury poisoning displays the same signs and symptoms in children who have been diagnosed with autism.

Chapter 5: Warnings from a chemist who created the vaccine

While people can choose to believe or not believe what the main stream media eagerly feeds them, one thing is for certain. When vaccinations were first created by a female chemist she tried them to heed her warnings when it came to injecting the body with these harmful substances. As both she and others have proven countless times, there is no substitute for what our bodies can do naturally.

Vaccinations don't work

The real truth

Not only have we learned of the deadly toxins including some that were claimed to no longer be used and still are, but we also have learned the truth and that is they don't work. We've heard it time and time again that science doesn't like and even more so from the mouth of our very own president. That's true to a certain degree. Science can't lie, people however, can and do. If we were to actually read the facts and the countless hours and centuries of research that is done, there is no real reason to vaccinate.

If we open our eyes and look beyond the money making chain of big pharmaceutical companies we could see that we are doing more harm than good. In addition, it has been proven through science time and time again that something lab made cannot do what our bodies do naturally. Several tests have been doing using primates to study the effects of vaccinations and how they would respond to or in our bodies. The results came in pretty clear, our bodies do better work naturally than by a forced chemical into our blood stream. When animal antibodies and other special components were used, it was noted that they had zero effect in protecting us and boosting immunity. Actually, quite the opposite seemed to be true in this case. When injected with animal antibodies along with these chemicals, were more susceptible to contracting the illness and thus spreading it to others.

The rise and fall of vaccinations

Dr. Maurice Hilleman

So who exactly is responsible for this whole vaccination epidemic anyway? The answer lies back in 1948. Here Mr. Hilleman became the chief of Respiratory Diseases. During this time Hong Kong who had been hit with an influenza epidemic after he worked hard and discovered some genetic changes after a mutation in the flu virus. After nine long days of hard work, both Hilleman and his colleague discovered just how deadly the virus was and a vaccination was quickly prepared and distributed.

In 1957, Hilleman joined Merck&Co. and became head of the virus and cell biology department. Here he developed over forty experimental and license vaccines that could be used on both animals and humans. In 1963 his daughter who caught mumps lead to the creation of the vaccine that he made. This later opened the door-way to the first ever live multi-strained virus created.

Remember some of those not so pleasant chemicals we mentioned earlier? After his creation of the Hepatitis B vaccine, one of the ingredients he used to combat this disease formaldehyde. Later this vaccine was withdrawn and replaced with a similar one that involved using Yeast instead. While in the creation of numerous vaccines it was Hilleman that warned that the simian virus might contaminate other vaccines which was used in the Polio vaccine.

Due to the contamination issues with the simian virus, the Polio virus was forced to be recalled in 1961 and replaced with an oral vaccine created by Albert Sabin. Ironically, both the oral and its previous form both were contaminated, but it was found that the oral vaccine did not produce any harm or issues unlike its counter-part form since it was ingested instead of injected.

Chapter 6: The dangers of multiple shots at one time for a child

Just about anywhere you go when it comes to vaccines you will notice that they give vaccinations in multiple doses at once. While they may spread out "series" of shots, they are still injecting children and newborns alike with different vaccinations in one visit. While some think it to be efficient or even "better" for the child involved there is a lot more harm involved than good. Here are some things to consider when you inject a single child with multiple vaccines at once:

What is the necessity that the child involved is having all these does at once?

How will my child benefit from multiple vaccinations per visit?

Is there a better way?

There has been zero proof that vaccinating children with multiple inoculations at once benefits them at all. In fact, there have been more issues involving multiple dosing's at once than anything else. Many parents have reported that directly after having their child vaccinated they experienced seizures, diagnosed with Autism, Asthma, Celiac disease, and these are just a few cases not including some of the side effects that are being passed off as "rare" or "Unusual" in terms of them happening.

Yet here we are still facing an extreme rise in Autism diagnosis's as well as children and babies being harmed by this "cultural norm." Eyes need to be opened and minds need to be widened so we can begin to understand the harm these chemicals and unnatural pollutants are having on the minds and bodies of our children. Unfortunately, it seems that once a parent brings their beliefs and findings about their child's distress post-vaccination they're quickly dismissed.

Of course everyone is going to deny they harmed an innocent child or baby over money, how else would they sleep well at night? We need stronger laws to protect our innocent and something better than just a phone number to call and inform a stranger that a child didn't respond well to a vaccination. There are more natural approaches that can be taken to ensure the health and safety of your child that don't need you putting chemicals and toxins in a body and are effective.

Homeopathic remedies

A new cure for an old problem
Many people, especially those who are pro-vaccine look down

on homeopathic remedies. Even when it comes to something as simple as trying to elevate your child's worst cold symptoms, pediatrician's alike snub their nose down at them. So while its seemingly okay to fill your child's body with dangerous toxins, it's apparently not okay to give them something natural that actually help safely, are cost effective and work better.

A new practice has started to sweep its way across the nations and that is "Nosodes." If this is a new term to you or you find yourself a skeptic just keep in mind while this is not a 'real' vaccination in terms of what your child may receive at the clinic or doctor, it is healthier, safer, and effective. After all, if we can spare our child not only the dangerous chemicals and not put their bodies at risk why not try a different alternative?

How do Nosodes work?

Short-term disease prevention

A nosode is just a small sample of a live virus. While typical vaccines work by putting "Dead virus" cells in the body (among other things) and expecting it to do the job of prevention, a nosode works in the opposite. A small strain of the live virus (Whichever is being attempted to be prevented), and injected just the same. The only difference is there is nothing else in the vaccine. There are no additives, there is no mercury or any other harmful substances to be found in it.

How does it work?

Knowing if Nosodes are right for you

While this may not be ideal for every parent there are currently no known side effects and no death or injuries as a result. The dose given is so small that while it allows the body to fight it off naturally, it also recognizes the virus and builds the immunity without the side effects. In some parts of the world such as France, they have been known to have out breaks of the measles. While some parents may not want to rush to the vaccine clinic or may not have ever vaccinated their child before, this is a healthy alternative.

A parent can locate their local Homeopath in their area that specializes in this area of expertise and then they get a dose and are protected for a few weeks at a time. To some this may seem pointless since it doesn't provide long-term protection, however, it does allow the body to recognize the virus in the future if they come in contact and the body now knows how to fight it off and it no longer becomes an issue of immunity. Nosodes are even ideal for those who enjoy traveling. If you plan on going to an area who may have an outbreak or an epidemic of a certain disease then you can get your vaccination for it and be protected along with future prevention already stored in your body.

Perhaps the best part about this approach is not only is it

chemical free and there are no side-effects, but you're teaching your body how to fight off diseases in a more natural way. There is no risk of Autism, there is no risk of death, and there is no risk of any side effect that you would find in a typical vaccine. It's a new age approach that works. Of course there will always be skeptics and people who can't believe that something so simple works or could be effective, but many people in Europe are definitely giving a thumbs up to a healthy new alternative for their children.

Chapter 7: The Ingredients in the vaccines

My vaccine has what?

For those that choose to vaccinate, you will notice that they willingly accept the hype created about them as eagerly as they do the lies that come with inoculations. While they have sit back and hungrily ate up the lies the media spits out for them to hear, they have failed to realize what tiny part; the compound of a vaccine. On any given day if you walk in to a doctor's office or a vaccination clinic you will be unlikely to ever hear a parent ask what exactly is in the vaccination's given to their children.

In fact usually it's just a signed piece of paper, a quick ramble of the usual information provided and a few pokes for your child. The visit is over, you leave and that's the end of that until the next round of shots are due to be administered. What if I told you though, that there are some hidden culprits inside that vaccine, which was more than just a "dormant virus" bonding with your child's body as a way of creating antibodies and immunity against something they'll probably never get anyway?

If we were to break down a vaccine in to its smaller components we'd see that beyond a virus it contains a lot more than what meets the eye. Things that aren't discussed in news articles, medical journals or even the mess that comes from the television consistently. No, there is something sinister just sitting and waiting to be unleashed and once it has the effects are neither pleasant nor irreversible.

If you were to ask a physician the components of a vaccine you'd probably get quite a strange look. It's also possible you'd hear something similar to "Saline, sterile water, and preservatives containing protein." Luckily, we'll do your homework for you and take a look into the ingredients that nobody talks about. First and foremost, you will always find two major components:

-Mercury

-Thermosil (There's your "protein preservative"

Of course I'm sure the others listed are there too but not nearly as important as these two...but let's keep going...

-Aluminum

- Amino Acids and Proteins

-Formaldehyde

-Benzethonium Chloride

-Glutaraldehyde

-MSG

-CTMB

-Phenoxyethanol

I really want to take a look further in to some of these ingredients so that everyone understands the risk that they pose and exactly what their "purpose" is in the big scheme of things. So, let's start from the top and we'll work our way down the list accordingly.

-Aluminum: Just about everything around us contains traces of this chemical and said to be harmless if swallowed or breathed in the small amounts that we do daily. It has to be harmless then right? Wrong, even though it's used to make vaccines "work better," anyone who had real medical knowledge would understand the risks involved when injected in to the body. Anyone who allows this to be injected in their bodies is receiving more than the recommended amount and have been shown to demonstrate illness related to those with nervous system and bone toxicity. Newborns are especially high risk for this type of issue.

-Amino Acids and Proteins: Surely this must be a good thing right? After all it's what our body is composed of. Wrong again. When injected in to the body and combined with the vaccine amino acids and proteins respond a bit differently. They turn in to antigens (the vaccine) which is made to trigger the immune system and get them to learn how to fight off invasive illness and diseases. In this case however, it tricks your body and causes it to respond in not such positive ways. Some of those include autoimmune disorders such as Addison's disease, Celiac Disease, Graves' disease, diabetes and food sensitive's and allergies just to name a few.

-Formaldehyde: I think we are all a little bit too familiar with its typical purpose in preserving things especially when it comes to a loved, but deceased family member or friend. So what exactly could its role play in vaccinations? Unbeknownst to many it's a toxic that causes cancer. If injected with too high of a dose it's known to cause nerve damage, death, flu or cold like symptoms, ear aches, depression, loss of red blood cells and the list goes on.

-Benzethonium Chloride: This one is a bit strange and probably one of the biggest kept secrets when it comes to vaccine ingredients. While there is little information to be found (or easily), it does suggest that it's hazardous if inhaled, injected as well to human skin. Yet here we are injecting vaccines readily into our skin AND body. Another big leading problem that can cause cancer. Side effects include seizures, coma, respiratory depression, Central Nervous System Depression, Convulsions, and Urinary tract reaction. Very little research has been done on this ingredient, but yet were okay to include this in to a vaccine and place in to our children's bodies.

-Glutaraldehyde: Another chemical that is found to be iffy at best. Typically this ingredient is used in sterilizing medical equipment, but is used as a preservative in vaccinations. Side effects include: Asthma, Allergic reactions, diarrhea, and induced respiratory issues.

-Thermisol: Need we say more? Preservative that includes mercury and we all know what that can do.

-Yeast Extract/MSG: This is by far one of the more surprising ingredients. With a vast amount of people allergic to MSG, Dairy or have a yeast allergy this would naturally make a vaccination dangerous. Side effects can include: Allergic reaction, Seizure, Stroke, Diabetes, Alzheimer's, IBS and more. The egg protein as mentioned above is highly dangerous to those who have an allergy to eggs, dairy and so forth.

-CTMB: Another chemical labeled as hazardous, and is an irritant to just about every part of the human body. Not only that it's harmful to fish and flammable. Any information about this suggests that it should not be consumed in any form or manner and in doing so should seek medical help immediately. With that being said, anyone near or handling this dangerous chemical is ordered to wear special safety material handling gear. Symptoms may not show up for several hours and can continue up to 48 hours after ingestion.

-Phenoxyethanol: Antibacterial agent in vaccines, toxic to

swallow and otherwise harmful and an irritant to the body. Issues with this vary from genetic mutations to reproductive issues, and anything from death, cardiac/kidney failure, weakness, and convulsions among other things.

Most people are blind and uniformed of these very specific type of chemicals found in the vaccines that they load their children up on. If people were more informed the rate of vaccines would dramatically drop and of course that means major pharmaceutical companies would go out of business, but out government can't have that. Perhaps, the saddest part of all is that many parents provided this information, would still willingly and knowingly inject their children with it anyway to save from a threat that is unlikely to ever occur.

Chapter 8: Dangers of mercury in the brain

Some of the ways the human body is affected when mercury is injected happen not only in the body systems, but the organs as well. Issues with the immune system, cardiovascular system, neurological, gastrointestinal as well as kidneys and liver have all been known to be affected. At least ten percent of neonates have been exposed to mercury levels while in womb that is greater than what the FDA considers "Safe." When unsafe levels of mercury are present in a person's system, it seems to almost destroy their immune system or at the very least impair it. In some findings, children who were diagnosed with autism demonstrated the same behaviors and effects as those with mercury poisoning. Some of these symptoms include: psychiatric disturbances, speech and language issues, hearing problems, unusual behavior, sensory abnormalities, and cognitive impairment. Mercury however, isn't the only known toxin found inside vaccines. While Thimerosal and mercury are an issue, aluminum has also been found inside vaccines and played a major role as well.

It almost seems ironic for mercury to be found in a vaccine. After all, it's known to lower a child's IQ and thus make them less economically productive over a life time. Keep the masses ignorant to what goes on around them or what's being put in to things they consume and they won't think to ask questions. If people are made ignorant to what they consume then nobody is going to know better and nobody is going to raise a fuss about the harmful things that they're ingesting or in this case injecting in to their body or those of their children.

Some of our major medical mysteries can actually link back to mercury, the effect it has on the human brain and some of the ailments that people are suffering in vast numbers across the globe today. Autism, ADHD, memory loss, Dementia, Alzheimer's Dementia and lack of focus have all linked back to exposure to mercury. With this being the case, it's safe to say the same issues people are reporting post- vaccination are strongly correlated despite what some may have you to believe.

Dementia is a brain dysfunction in which a person loses the ability to think, remember, reason and in most cases interferes with their everyday lives. In the world today, there are an estimated 24 million people with dementia worldwide. By 2040 it is estimated that number will rise severely to 81 million. While there are many causes behind Dementia/Alzheimer's Dementia one of the number one causes is mercury toxicity. Further research indicates that those suffering have higher levels of mercury than typical brains. Some adverse reactions to mercury toxicity (poisoning) are: tremors, impaired vision/hearing, paralysis, insomnia, emotional instability, developmental defects (in womb), and ADD during childhood.

Chapter 9: The explosion of cancer

Cancer is a growing epidemic that we are hearing more and more about these days. It seems to not only just be just affecting adults anymore, but we are not hearing more and more cases of childhood and newborn cases of cancer. One of the biggest stories involving cancer related injuries due to vaccines happened from the 1955-1963. The CDC admitted to tainting the polio virus with Simian Virus 40 (SV40) and because of this it is estimated that anywhere from between 10-30 million Americans were infected with the infected vaccine and are likely to have contracted cancer as a result.

Not surprisingly enough the US healthcare's major cash flow comes not only from vaccines, but cancer treatment and therapies. It only makes sense then that they want to force not only vaccines on us, but vaccines that contain cancer causing contaminants. We've all seen the commercials with young teens on them, mostly females advertising a vaccine to protect from HPV (human papilloma virus). Its intent is supposed to prevent cervical cancer/ovarian cancer in young women.

Unfortunately the opposite seems to be happening and in most cases, actually causes the virus to be entered in to the body and cause females to be contracting cancer. Not only is it's causing cancer, but it's also causing STD's such as genital warts to occur. Some other known side effects as a result of this "necessary" vaccination is head and neck tumors that are cancerous as well as dental cancers that form in the mouth, larynx, and nasal cavities among others.

Tongue and tonsillar cancer make up the most common type associated with this vaccine and often develop together inside the body. Usually, only five percent of patients diagnosed with tongue and tonsillar cancer survive and require extensive therapies and medicines just to treat, manage and bring the patient comfort until the inevitable where it steals their lives.

While this trend has been on the rise for the last number of years due to the vaccine, the CDC has attempted to shift the blame from both them and the FDA to the actual patients themselves. How can a child be responsible for causing cancer, let alone knowingly? Well according to the CDC it's not the vaccine that strictly causes these types of cancer with a high mortality rate, but the sexual activities of the teens themselves. That's right, by engaging in oral sex, or open-mouth kissing (French kissing), and vaginal intercourse you are causing and raising the risk of getting cancer.

I don't know about anyone else, but if sexual intercourse and fore-play was the leading cause of cancer it seems to me that almost everyone in the world who was not a virgin should be dying of cancer right now. The truth remains in the ingredients that are placed in our vaccines. It doesn't matter if you are sleeping with just one partner or your sleeping around, vaccines are the cause to most of our health problems in our youth and adults today. We learned in health class growing up and from our doctors that if you had multiple partners the end result was pregnancy or possibility of an STD/VD. Now we have physicians telling us to safe-guard our children with vaccines to prevent cancer, when in turn it's causing our kids to get worse cancer then they may have ever been at risk for to begin with.

While Dr. Hilleman was a leading pioneer in the creation of over three-dozen vaccinations he was also the one who tried to warn so many about the dangers including that of cancer. Before his untimely death years later, Hilleman was interviewed and reported that not only did he take responsibility for the spread of cancer due to the contamination via the Polio virus, but that it was in the same way that people were likely suffering from AIDS. In 2002 it was discovered and published that almost every case involving non-Hodgkin lymphoma cases were a result of the infected vaccinations from the simian virus.

As a result more than sixty studies in a lab confirmed that in almost every case of bone, brain, lung and lymphatic cancer the presence of SV40 was found by researcher Dr. Michele Carbone. It was during the years 1953-1963 that evidence began to turn up compelling evidence that the infected virus was causing tumors in those who had received the vaccination for Polio and was still showing up in tests in children who were born in 1983. What this means is that years after this vaccination had been altered and the simian virus removed, trace evidence was being passed down genetically through blood lines and quite possibly still in existence within the vaccinations people were receiving. Many scientists believed that not only had they not removed the virus in vaccinations despite warnings, but it was kept and continuously injected in to those receiving it until as late as 1999.

While after no other cases of polio were being reported as occurring as an effect of the inoculation from 1980-1999, there were an estimated 144 cases reported that were a direct cause of the oral vaccination. If receiving the virus via ingestion wasn't bad enough, further reports indicated that for those who had received the oral vaccination it was showing up in feces for up to two months and in the throat for two weeks post-vaccination which meant that it was spreadable to others who had not received the vaccination at all.

Once more in 1999 the Polio virus was reformulated, this time to contain a "dead" version of the virus, although there have been reports and side effects that have come with this version as with the rest too. Much like with the Polio virus, it has been found that more cases of cancer surfaced in young females and women inoculated with the HPV virus. However, it recent studies it has also been proven that young boys have also fallen victim to other forms of cancer too.

Chapter 10: People dropping like flies (Dying)

So if you haven't been convinced by now why you shouldn't vaccinate your children let's look at some scary statistics. You see, other than pressing our government to enforce stronger and safer laws about our vaccines and what goes in them we can't do much about the dangerous chemicals or what goes with it. What we can do however, is be prepared to make a choice and a stance about our children and their lives. It's not just the side-effects of the chemicals you have to worry about, it's not just about the possibility of cancer, and it's about possibly never seeing your child again.

You see the mortality rate of newborns and infants are on the rise. Years ago we were introduced to SIDs. As far as new parents were concerned or even those who had children before, SIDs was the only scary illness that were going to take their children from them. New studies suggest however, that nations that require more vaccines for babies had a higher mortality rate than those who did not.

For whatever reason, the United States requires more vaccines for newborns than anybody else (26). Due to this, for every 6+ babies that are born alive and well, 1,000 will never live to take their first steps, say their first words or ever see the light of day. In fact, some infant death cases (SIDs) are actually due to vaccines or over vaccination. In that sense it's like playing Russian roulette with your child's life. You never know if the next vaccine you administer is the last one they will ever get or if it will be the last time you ever see them alive again.

While studies in the past deny the correlation behind infant related deaths and vaccines, you can't deny there is definitely a link. To view the past evidence including, the chemicals, the side effects and then babies dying "mysteriously" after being injected with these chemicals there is no denying the truth. Vaccines are a danger to everyone both young and old. Young females are passing away due to cancers that certain vaccines are supposed to prevent. The chemicals and toxins inside the vaccinations including two main components are linked to having caused cancer. People are dying constantly and I don't think it's by mere coincidence.

It's easy for a health official or our government to blame it on society or to blame it on living conditions ("other factors"). The bottom line is you can't just blame a person's life on their illness or their death. There are plenty of places in the world where people DO have drinkable water that is safe, they DO have the means to live and support a healthy lifestyle. However, when you introduce something like this, it's only natural that people are going to start dropping dead left and right because of an unsafe factor that is being included in to their bloodstream and lives.

Chapter 11: The statistics now compared to the seventies

For anyone who has grown up in the seventies in comparison to today's world, they'll all agree that a lot has changed. Not just the technology, but general health as a whole. Vaccines in the seventies weren't as common as it was still something new then. The CDC even goes to explain that vaccines then were protecting people from seven different diseases compared to the sixteen we are "prevented" from today.

Unfortunately, with these changes came a lot of health concerns and problems as well. Some children legitimately do have certain illnesses that may require medication to control so they can live a normal life. There are far more however, that do not require medication and are being slapped with a label just so they can be profited from. Let's take a look at a few of these in further detail and get a better look at just how far we've come, or perhaps how much we've stepped back.

Currently ADD/ADHD is one of the largest over-diagnosed and medicated example. In the seventies they would label a child diagnosed with this disease as being "hyper" or just needing to get outside more. Now we find that 11% of children ranging in ages from 4 years old to seven years old have been diagnosed with ADD. In the seventies it was not much different, however, how we handled things were. Children who are younger and within Kindergarten age ranges are about 60% more likely to be placed on some form of medication and diagnosed with ADD.

Another large difference is during the seventies people still believed that a doctor and medicine could fix all their ailments. They were not concerned with disease or vaccinations unlike today where as they are pushed upon everyone. Ironically, the CDC claims they have zero laws in place that "force" or require any person to get a vaccination, but each state does. There were possibly twelve total vaccines a child of the seventies received and yet by the year 2013, the CDC, AAFP and AAP have endorsed children to have over 36 vaccinations by the time they turned six years of age.

So instead of just a few "necessary" vaccines to protect our children, they were forced to be pumped full of thirty six different vaccinations each with potent and harmful chemicals. Nobody thought to question vaccinations around the seventies because there was no substantial amount of information or research made available to the public to become more aware of what they were putting in to their children. We also weren't aware of the back room deals where pharmaceutical companies were being paid to lie about the effects on children or the supposed "necessity" of these inoculations.

If that wasn't alarming enough, let's compare some mortality rates to show just how much difference there is between not only the amount of required inoculations and the effect it's having. In 1992, a study was done and showed that children were 8% more likely to die than normal after having the DPT vaccination. Children who had another "necessary" vaccination called HiB were five times more likely to contract the disease than those who didn't get the vaccination and that 80% of children who have been vaccinated against whooping cough got it opposed to those who went unvaccinated.

In 1977 a German scientist responsible for the creation of the Polio vaccination testified with many others like himself, and announced that almost 90% of cases of polio that occurred in the United States since the 1970's was a direct result of the vaccination itself. So here we have another example of scientists who created these vaccines telling people the dangers of what can happen and warning that in most cases you either wind up with the disease its mean to prevent or in other cases death. Currently, the polio vaccine is the only "known" cause of the polio disease today in the United States.

In 1980 the American Medical Associate noted that 90% of both pediatricians and obstetricians refused to take the rubella vaccine. If a doctor is refusing to take a vaccination that the general public is being "required" to take then something doesn't quite add up correctly here. Vaccinations we are being told are meant to help us are worrying and hurting enough people that even doctors at that point refused them. What does that say to you?

Chapter 12: Preventive Measures

How can I protect my family?

So, most have the same thoughts on their mind when it comes to vaccinations, or at least those who are anti-vaccination. How can I protect my family? Some states vary in laws and regulations when it comes to vaccinations. Certain doctor's offices may require a simple waiver form saying that you acknowledge they want your child to be vaccinated as well as your refusal. Nobody wants their child sick or hurt and there are always certain steps that can be taken to prevent this.

If you're unsure about your states statutes and laws regarding vaccinations feel free to talk to your pediatrician, law-enforcement officer or state board health to ask questions and learn more about what your options are. One such choice to vaccinate your child and get around injecting them with chemicals and toxins are trying the homeopathic approach. As mentioned in a previous chapter it is more natural and the only thing your child receives is a significantly small sample of the virus which their body fights off naturally without any adverse side-effects.

Other possibilities depending on the virus is natural

immunization through contact. This simply means in cases such as the flu and chicken pox (both inoculations the CDC backs) allow the child to receive direct contact with a person infected. While nobody wants to have either of these nasty illnesses, allowing your child to get the flu or chicken pox is one way of boosting natural immunity without the requirement of a vaccination. From times as early as the 50's on forward, parents use to send their kids to neighbors and family members homes who had children with the chicken pox virus. By allowing them to play together and contract the virus they in turn infected their own children but allowed them a natural immunity where in most cases the child never contracted the virus again.

Vitamin's for some diseases are also a plus. While certain vaccinations do have flu-like or cold-like symptoms afterwards, vitamins can help aid in the healing part of this. Centuries ago when pirates were more popular and known to ravage the seas, scurvy was a big issue. They didn't create a vaccine for this, instead oranges was the solution. Much like today, we can pick up over the counter (OTC) medications that help boost immunity to certain illnesses and promote well-being.

Other easy tips to disease prevention that most vaccinations claim they prevent is to be mindful of your area. If you don't tend to travel abroad then it's extremely unlikely that you're going to pick up some of the diseases that are supposed to be prevented. Most diseases that are preventable are not contagious minuses cases such as the cold, flu or chicken pox.

Chapter 13: Detoxing out these heavy metals

So let's say that you are pro-vaccine or that you just don't feel comfortable with not vaccinating your child, what can you do about those nasty toxins and chemicals they've just entered in to your child? There have been many proven methods of detoxing your body from pollutants or other potentially harmful chemicals. Maybe you've vaccinated your child and you want to rid of the heavy metals, or maybe you want to and just want your child safe. Either way, we are going to take a look in to some steps on how to remove these nasty toxins for a happier, healthier and safer child.

For some parents who are okay with vaccinations there are mercury free based vaccinations that are available. The first step in removing chemicals that are harmful is eating well. I know it sounds a little cliché and like something you would hear out of a dietary commercial but it's true. Your biggest goal is to eat as many vegetables (Didn't your mother warn you to eat your veggies?) and avoid sugar and manufactured goods that are processed or refined.

The second step is you have to work on fixing your immune system. While vitamins are helpful, you need a much stronger approach. Sugars are found in the vaccines that you get and are quite harmful to the body since they suppress the immune system. Sugars are also known to feed parasites, fungus, bacteria and other types of viruses looking to make us sick. While garlic is your best go to supplement by mixing these other ingredients in as well you'll be on the right track. Try adding these great supplementary foods to your diet: Oil of oregano, Echinacea, goldenseal, and goldthread. When used together they purify the blood, remove harmful toxins as well as repair the immune system.

Another great step is stocking up on Vitamin B rich foods and supplements. Drinking lots of fluids and exercising is another great key. I know that might strange, but believe it or not it's not much different than when you're sick. The healthier and better you eat and drink and stay fit the better your immune system works. Likewise in ridding of these toxins, you want to eat and drink and stay healthy and you'll have a better chance at detoxing from these toxins.

One thing to keep in mind is detoxing is supposed to be a slow and gentle process. Otherwise, it wouldn't be called detoxing. While I am in no way a doctor nor sponsored by one, there are right and wrong ways to go about these steps which are a lot of common sense too. While the above are some ways to detox an adult, detoxing a child is different and has to be done a lot gentler. Keep in mind that detoxing usually takes at least a month and depending on if you or your loved one has suffered an adverse reaction, it may take a little bit longer.

Detoxing heavy metals from my child

Safe detoxing and removal

Start with a detoxification bath. Typically, all children enjoy bath time whether due to splashing and bubbles or their favorite bath toy this is a great start. The detoxification bath is used to pull bacteria and viruses from the spine, and harmful chemicals and toxins from the body. By adding five drops of Purification Essential Oil with just a few sprinkles of high quality sea-salt you'll be on your way in no time. If your child is a bit older and will sit still you may also substitute with a foot bath using the same steps.

Probiotics are also another great way to go, they balance the immune system and is extremely helpful if your child experienced a negative reaction to the vaccine. The powdered form of "Life Start" is a great way to go and if your child has a dairy sensitivity there is also the option of a dairy free version of it.

Omega 3 Fish Oil no matter young or old is a great way to boost immunity and balance your immune system out as well. There are just a lot of great and natural ingredients that work for various parts of your body. For children you may consider finding one's that are free of the dreaded "Fish taste" that often comes with taking this supplement regularly.

This one is kind of a biggie when it comes to the detoxification process for a lot of reasons. Cilantro Chelation Therapy was discovered in the leaves of the coriander plant which accelerates the removal of mercury and aluminum from the body. Both gentle and inexpensive, Cilantro binds to the harmful chemicals and pulls them from your body. Please note do not use the pill form as its least effective and not bound to do a whole lot. However, you can eat raw or cook with it. Your child should get a minimum of one teaspoon 2-3 times a week or you may add to their bath and do a detox with salt as mentioned above in the detox bath article.

Elderberry, one of the best supplements for children and can be taken in syrup or supplement form. Research has shown that elderberries have inhibited enzymes and used by viruses to make you sick. Another form that is possible is Elderberry Defense which contains Echinacea, royal jelly and olive leaf. It strengthens the immune system, fights viral infections, and increases the production of T-lymphocytes which fights bacterial toxins.

The royal jelly contains nutrients found in all eight amino acids that help prevent illness. Olive leaf has been proven to remove almost every disease-causing microorganisms. Vitamin C as we mentioned earlier in the guide is a great way to go. It naturally boosts the immune system and can be found in many foods including oranges or in a chewable tablet form and gummies for younger children.

Silica gently removes toxins from your blood stream and tissues which allows your body to safely remove it. Research and studies show that it's one of the most effective ways to gently and safely, yet effectively remove aluminum from your body. It can be found in liquid form or as an herbal supplement.

As we mentioned previously, anything homeopathic is typically a great route to go and especially with children. If you have someone who specializes in these types of things in your area it's a great idea to consult with them and they can provide you with some other methods and ideas on what you can take or even safely give to your child to detox from a vaccination or reaction from receiving an inoculation.

Water seems to be typically great for just about everything and in this case it's really no different. Any time it comes to toxins and removing them you want to have them flushed from the body. In doing so water is the natural source for that. You want to avoid any sugar drinks and try to get your child to drink at least six to eight cups. For kids who aren't fond of the taste you can use honey or lemon to give it some flavor.

This one might seem a little funny but a good massage is the next step. No, really, you want to "milk the lymph nodes." The lymphatic system is a great part of the system that removes of waste. By massaging it you're helping to remove waste cells, proteins, excess fluids, viruses, and bacteria that get trapped there.

Dandelion Root is another key ingredient in the filtration process. We all know that the kidney serves to remove toxins from the body. However, when the toxins are heavier then we want to protect the liver as it works hard. Dandelion aids in this and is by far not only the safest but the most effective as well. While helping the liver it also helps the gallbladder to filter out the toxins, purify the blood and stimulates the kidneys to eliminate toxins through urine. This one is a bit of a freebie as you don't necessarily have to go to the store and purchase it, they grow naturally in your back yard.

Raw food and smoothies are a bit of a fun way to go. They counter attack the harmful effects of the vaccine and children love them. Ideally, you want them to drink about two or three of them a day included with a meal. Some of the best foods to use are broccoli, collards, radishes, onion, spices and sunny side up eggs. (Preferably from free-range chickens.)

Let the detoxing begin

Side-effects

Just like with any diet change or new regiment of medications there are always side-effects, but ideally they are a lot better than those of the vaccines and only temporary. Some of the things you may notice or they can experience are loose stools, grumpy for a few days, worsening symptoms (for those experiencing side effects from the vaccines), sleeping longer, possible flu-like symptoms, although children are less likely than adults to experience any side effects at all.

Once you've began this process it's really important to try and find a doctor or practitioner in your area to better address both your needs and those of your child to better help. A natural doctor or practitioner can better help to focus specifically on your needs of those and your child and target whatever effects you're suffering and offer help. If you're unable to locate one in your area the best thing you can do is "Juice out." This is a great way to deal with the toxicity issues as well as any deficiencies and is completely safe to do.

Keep in mind that when you do a detox it is at your own sole discretion and that I am in no way a doctor or trained physician. The methods described in this guide are suggestions and while none of this has been evaluated or approved by the FDA, each individual ingredient or suggestion has been recommended by homeopaths who specialize in this type of medicine and is by their recommendation the best alternative route to go to when vaccines are no longer the answer.

Chapter 14: Heavy Metals

If we've learned nothing else about vaccines, we have learned there are a lot of toxins and not so shockingly, heavy metals. As we've seen, mercury is by far one of those most common and dangerous one's that have been included. We've noted that in large doses and quantities it can make someone extremely sick or in some cases kill them.

In 2001, the CDC declared mercury to be toxic in all forms and dangerous to women, children and fetuses. The American Pediatrics recommended that while being unsafe it's in everyone's best interest that it be removed from the general population as far as exposure is concerned.

Mercury has been traced as far back as ancient Rome as a poison. Placed in to our vaccines since 1930's the results have always been roughly the same, cell injury and cell death. Beyond attacking our cells, mercury has been linked to destroying the central nervous system, brain damage and the onset of millions of cases of children being diagnosed with ADD and ADHD.

Vaccines aren't the only thing that we are exposed to containing mercury. Any time you have gone to the dentist and have gotten a filling it contained Mercury. Every time you have a filling you are filling your blood stream with more and more mercury. Unfortunately, mercury poisoning doesn't always show up right away and in some cases even takes decades. Amalgam fillings are a major contributing factor to people with brain damage cognitive dysfunction seen in elders.

That's not where it ends though. Anyone who was born in the 80's or earlier can probably remember getting sick and mom or dad taking their temperatures with thermometers. Unfortunately, if one of these broke you were directly ingesting a toxic level of mercury. Other everyday products have known to contain mercury as well including light bulbs.

If you thought mercury wasn't bad enough it's been shown that aluminum in vaccinations is by far worse. Aluminum is a well-known neurotoxin that is found in both adult and childhood vaccines and in some cases may exceed the toxicity of mercury in the human body. According to a study done in current medical chemistry, children up to six months of age are getting over 14.7 to 49 times more aluminum in vaccines than the FDA allows.

While the rise of people being against mercury based vaccines has grown, scientists have started to replace the mercury in them with aluminum. The process of aluminum in the vaccine was meant to boost your immune response. Through recent studies however, it has been found that aluminum has had no effect on the immune system and thus is doing more harm than good.

While aluminum has been found in just about everything from our air, to our soil and water that doesn't mean it's safe or natural. Aluminum has found to serve no biological role inside the body and instead is extremely poisonous and harmful. In fact, it has been associated with autoimmunity issues, long-term brain inflammation and other neurological complications. Other such disorders that have been identified as a direct result are multiple sclerosis, Alzheimer's disease, Parkinson's and ALS.

Often times when your child receives a vaccination the aluminum much like with mercury does not simply just enter the blood stream, but travels to the brain and accumulates there. The American Pediatrics Association has now admitted that aluminum is being implicated in causing major issues with the cellular structure, metabolic processes in the nervous systems and other tissues. Furthermore, it makes it harder for the body to remove mercury and whatever amount of mercury your body may contain is now being intensified.

One way to get rid of aluminum is retaining enough sulfur in your body. The reason for this being so essential is it's a powerful detoxifier and can help to expel these harmful chemicals from the body. While vaccinations have been around for a better part of ninety years, there are still very loose rules and regulations pertaining to them and even more so there doesn't seem to be any in the works.

Conclusion

top until our voices have been heard. There are so many alternatives to what we are injecting in our bodies today. If people from centuries past survived without these so called "miracle" cures then why can't wln short there is no right or wrong way to be a parent. So many people are focused on labeling one another as a good or bad parent based on their choices regarding their children. Many feel that for those who choose to be anti-vaccine that they are confused, poor informed or haven't done the proper research. The same goes for those that choose to vaccinate, many call them sheep, poorly educated or blind to what is lying right in front of them.

Instead of tearing each other down, parents need to be coming together and realizing a few things. First and foremost, our government is not going to tell you the truth. When most of their major source of income comes from those being sick, they aren't going to be quick to provide a healthy and safe cure or temporary fix to a medical problem. Think in terms of cancer. We spend millions upon millions of dollars to research this disease, cures and medicines to fix it.

Yet, almost every vaccination that we hand out has a direct link to causing cancer or cancer components. In turn this means that the same people who are paid to do the research are helping major pharmaceutical companies to become even wealthier by rolling out cures and "fix all's" to make someone feel better.

Just about every ailment we have ever seen or experienced you can guarantee there is a commercial in which there is always a pill for. Unfortunately, however, just like with vaccines, the end results are always worse than the actual issue. Remember those awful commercials that use to air about the sick baby with whooping cough?

They were always so heart-breaking and sad. You see this poor helpful newborn coughing and so sick. The narrator comes on and explains that how by not being vaccinated you've caused this poor defenseless newborn to pass away from an illness that could have been prevented had you just gotten you and your family inoculated. What they don't of course tell you is people who actually get a vaccine are the ones who get this vaccine and pass it on to others instead of the other way around.

Had they told the truth there would have been no money to be made. Do you suffer from depression, anxiety, pain? Well you're in luck because there is a pill like that. Even more of these commercials flash across our screen on a daily basis attempting to sell us some kind of pill that will be a magical cure-all for whatever ailment or mental illness you're experiencing.

The next thing you know a narrator comes on and quickly fires off information about how this can cause death, seizures, strokes, and cancer or suicidal thoughts. That's what vaccinations have in common with these same commercials, they want you to buy in to something that is supposed to be preventive or a fix to everyday problems with little regards to what may happen.

If the FDA told us that we were better off risking our life and taking chances with ourselves as we are then the pharmaceutical companies would have nothing to gain and nobody to make money off of. Likewise, they use tactics such as bullying and guilt to get us to do what they want. Some people are afraid to refuse a **vac**cine on the belief that they will lose their children due to medical neglect.

I'm not saying it hasn't happened, but I am saying that you have the right to stand up and choose what is right and what is wrong for your children. If you want to be pro-vaccine I won't knock you for it. You're standing up as a voice for your child to say you feel that the chemicals and side-effects that may happen as a direct result are better than the alternative. If you're like myself and many others and you feel that vaccines are not worth it then don't be afraid to stand up proudly and say the same. It's so easy for people to say they don't believe in something that isn't harmful to anyone (Breast feeding in public for example), but they're afraid to say they don't believe in something.

It's easy for people to say "I don't want my kids around someone who isn't vaccinated," then why is it not okay for someone to say "I don't want my kids around someone who is vaccinated because they're at risk." Kids are not informed of what's being put in to their bodies, but we have the ability to be informed and proactive. If more people stand up and say "That's not okay," then more laws and regulations that are much stricter can be put in to place and help keep our children from being exposed to these toxins and chemicals.

While I agree that not every child responds the same to vaccinations, it is unarguable that in some way or another it will eventually affect your child. Maybe they go for their regular set of twelve month vaccinations, they cry a little but otherwise wind up okay. Then fifty to sixty years down the line they develop a mental illness such as Alzheimer's Dementia with no prior family history. Maybe some can argue that as coincidence and maybe it is, but isn't it equally as plausible that something unnatural in a vaccination caused it too?

As parents we need to band together, teach each other and teach your children what goes in to these vaccinations. Open their eyes to what the media would like us to ignore and believe is false. Remember, we have been warned for generations from those who created these vaccinations from the start that they are not healthy or natural. After all, who really wants to inject a child with not only chemicals and toxins but parts of animal's organs and aborted fetuses? Even if you're pro-vaccine, surely you can't be okay with taking a baby that was brutally removed from a mother's womb and then altered and placed in to your child's body.

There is so much information to be found in medical journals. Doctors have always spouted off that we need vaccinations, but consider this as well....anyone who is paid to get you to do something that financially benefits another can't be a good thing. A doctor makes money by seeing patients, in turn if the can convince you to get a vaccination for something or to take a certain medication they are making money for those same pharmaceutical companies that are hurting you.

So the same company that made your prescription has now caused some sort of long-term illness which requires more visits to the doctor and thus it becomes a life cycle that continues. Inoculations are a lot like that too. You're sick so that must mean you need to be vaccinated. Now that you have received your vaccine you're sick. This means another trip to the doctor, more shots and maybe other types of medication or possible hospitalization. As this cycle continues to loop around and around your making a company who sleeps well at night knowing they've deceived the general public, into getting more and more medication and pills and making them money beyond imagination.

I will not blame someone for wanting to do better for themselves or their children. Much like you, I want what's best for my child. I want them to be happy, healthy and live active lives and watch their dreams come true. That's a natural desire for every parent for their children. Maybe some people don't have the means to educate themselves on the dangers of vaccinations. Maybe some have had it drilled in to their heads from the time of early understanding. We grew up asking our parents "why. Why do I have to do this" or "Why do I have to do that?" and the answer has always been "because I said so."

So are we now in an age of making excuses, where you have to suffer, you have to get this vaccination not because it's necessary, but because I said so. That's not good enough, educate yourself if you love your children. If you value your life, then educate yourself.

To each parent it is their choice and their personal business as to how they choose to raise their children. I will never tear a parent down for the life choices they make for their children as I would never want it to be done to me. However, I will always be the voice of reason and inform anyone who will listen what it means to vaccinate. I will teach my children as they grow older that it's not necessary. That their children and grandchildren can be healthy and happy and grow just fine without these chemicals introduced to their bodies.

I will allow them to make their own informed choices and if that's not enough, I will allow them to look for their own answers in a world full of knowledge. We can't force our views on other people, but we can point them in the right direction. So the next time you are in a doctor's office or with fellow mommy's, don't be afraid to speak up and help them to learn about the choices they made. You don't have to be forceful, but you can express yourself.

For too long our government has gotten away with us sitting by idly while we lose our children to allergic reactions to chemicals and compounds found inside of these vaccines. For far too long we have watched our children suffer through sicknesses and ailments that last anywhere from days to for the unfortunate few, a life time. By becoming pro-active, sign petitions, and spreading the world around we can take back our bodies and the right that we have.

Send a letter to the mayor's office, don't be afraid to se? It doesn't take much to understand that almost all vaccines that were getting and injecting our bodies with, are prevent diseases that are no longer in existence. By banding together with each other, we can make a difference and make a change.